Chest Pain

Chest Pain

Richard C. Becker, M.D.

Professor of Medicine,
University of Massachusetts Medical School, Worcester;
Director, Coronary Care Unit,
Cardiovascular Thrombosis Research Center,
and Anticoagulation Services,
UMass Memorial Medical Center,
Worcester

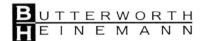

Boston Oxford Auckland Johannesburg Melbourne New Delhi

Recognizing the importance of preserving what has been written, Butterworth–Heinemann prints its books on acid-free paper whenever possible.

 Butterworth–Heinemann supports the efforts of American Forests and the Global ReLeaf program in its campaign for the betterment of trees, forests, and our environment.

Library of Congress Cataloging-in-Publication Data
Becker, Richard C.
    Chest pain / Richard C. Becker.
        p. cm. -- (The most common complaints)
    Includes bibliographical references and index.
    ISBN 0-7506-7141-6 (alk. paper)
1. Chest pain. 2. Angina pectoris. 3. Coronary heart disease. I. Title. II. Series.
RC941 .B39 2000
616.1'2--dc21   99-087184

British Library Cataloguing-in-Publication Data
A catalogue record for this book is available from the British Library.

The publisher offers special discounts on bulk orders of this book.
For information, please contact:
Manager of Special Sales
Butterworth–Heinemann
225 Wildwood Avenue
Woburn, MA 01801-2041
Tel: 781-904-2500
Fax: 781-904-2620

For information on all
Butterworth–Heinemann
publications available,
contact our World Wide Web
home page at:
http://www.bh.com

10 9 8 7 6 5 4 3 2 1

Printed in the United States of America

Dedicated to my parents, Ruth and Charles Becker,
my brother, Charlie, and my sister, Lynne,
who inspired my lifelong unconditional quest for knowledge.

Contents

PART THREE:
EVALUATION OF CHEST PAIN

PART FOUR:
MANAGEMENT OF ISCHEMIC
CHEST PAIN

PART FIVE:
CASE STUDIES

Tables

Preface

The clinician's approach to the diagnosis and management of chest pain is a journey that begins with a comprehensive understanding of anatomy and physiology and ends with the applied knowledge of pharmacology and treatment modalities based on carefully conducted clinical trials. The greatest challenge for the clinician lies in an existing vast array of pathobiologic entities that cause chest pain and the humbling range of clinical expressions for these processes, with fatal acute myocardial infarction on one end of the spectrum and universally benign but troubling conditions like costochondritis on the other. Despite the complexity and importance of making the correct diagnosis, it remains as clear today as it was during Sir William Osler's time that the approach to chest pain must directly involve the patient and follow a stepwise and orderly path if success is to be realized and optimal patient care is to be rendered—the ultimate goal in medicine and all clinical endeavors.

Chest Pain was written by a clinician for clinicians and is designed to meet the challenges and rapid evolution of in-hospital and ambulatory-based medical practice.

R.C.B.

Pain: Fundamental Concepts

Pain

A feeling of distress, suffering, agony.

A localized physical suffering caused by a bodily disorder.

A basic bodily sensation induced by a noxious stimulus that is experienced or perceived as uncomfortable or distressing.

Types of Pain

Pain, with little question, is the most common symptom or complaint for which patients seek medical attention. To comprehensively manage pain, the clinician must understand its origin, how it is perceived, and what, if any, influencing factors are involved. At a certain level, the clinician must, in essence, "feel what the patient is feeling" to determine the severity and urgency of the moment, yet remain objective to guide appropriate diagnostic testing and treatment.

The goals of management are twofold: first, to discover the etiology; and second, to treat the symptoms and clinical manifestations (even if the cause is not readily identifiable). It must be emphasized, however, that the initial focus must be on understanding the *cause* of pain.

Pain can be classified temporally as *acute* or *chronic*, physiologically as *somatic* or *visceral*, and causally as *medical* or *psychogenic*.[1]

Patients with severe *acute pain* often provide a clear description of its time of onset, character, and location. Frequently, there are objective associated findings on the physical examination that shed light on the origin and whether the symptoms represent a serious or potentially life-threatening problem.

Pain lasting more than several months is usually considered *chronic*. Among patients with chronic pain, the timing, character, and localization are often more vague and the psychological, social, and functional factors weigh heavily into overall clinical expression.

Somatic pain is caused by peripheral nerve activation and can be either sharp or dull in character. In most cases, somatic pain is well-localized and intermittent.

Visceral pain is caused by activation of visceral (nociceptive) receptors and most often is characterized as aching or cramping in quality.

Medical pain occurs in patients with physiologic or structural disease and is characterized by prolonged periods of pain alternating with pain-free periods or by unremitting pain that waxes and wanes in severity.

Psychogenic pain occurs without a structural or physiologic basis. In most instances, the symptoms are vague and do not correspond to a specific anatomic site. A psychiatric disorder often is known or suspected.

Psychophysiologic pain represents a unique situation where structural disease is present (or at least a past history of structural disease) but coexisting psychologic factors have an impact on the perception and expression of symptoms. A majority of patients spend considerable time thinking about or openly discussing their pain, often leading to "chronic illness behavior," social isolation, and dependency on narcotics or other medications (to which they rarely respond completely). This group of patients is the most difficult to evaluate and manage and, in many cases, extensive diagnostic testing is carried out, yielding unremarkable or inconclusive results.

REFERENCES

1. Marskey H, Bogdok N (eds). Classification of Pain: Descriptions of Chronic Pain Syndromes and Definition of Pain Terms. Report by the International Association for the Study of Pain Task Force on Taxonomy (2nd ed). Seattle: IASP Press, 1994.

CHAPTER TWO

The Neurology of Pain

Mechanical, chemical, or thermal threats to tissue integrity cause nociceptive neurons to increase their discharge rate. In acute pain, the intensity of nerve stimulation must surpass a threshold level for neuronal discharge to occur. The physiology of chronic pain differs slightly because sensitized nociceptors have an increased rate of basal (nonstimulated) discharge, a lowering of the stimulus threshold above which nerve firing rate increases, and a supranormal increase in discharge rate with each increase in stimulus strength.[1]

The nerve receptors themselves are activated by mediators (*ligands*) released from nearby damaged tissue, from the circulation, or from adjoining nerve endings (Figure 2-1).

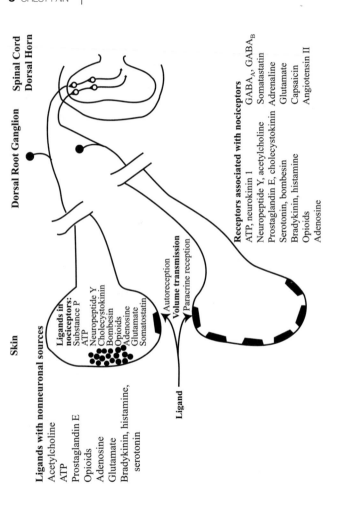

Figure 2-1. Nociceptive input is modified and integrated in the periphery. Receptors on nociceptive primary afferent fibers are activated by mediators released from nearby damaged tissue, from the circulation, or from the same or adjoining neurons. (Adapted with permission from SM Carlton, RE Coggeshall. Nociceptive integration: does it have a peripheral component? Pain Forum 1998;7:71–78.)

LOCALIZATION OF PAIN

In general, pain localizes over the site of origin and follows an orderly distribution determined by the autonomic nervous system (Figure 2-2). A cutaneous "map" (*dermatomes*) allows further localization; however, it is important to recognize that there is considerable overlap between adjacent dermatomes (Figure 2-3). In addition, there is overlap of sensory (*afferent*) nerve distribution among visceral organs, helping to explain the basis for "referred pain."

PERCEPTION OF CHEST PAIN

Chest pain perception is influenced strongly by several noncardiac and nonvisceral factors including age, race, gender, social class status, and comorbid illnesses such as diabetes mellitus, end-stage kidney disease, or cerebrovascular disease, particularly with one or more prior strokes. Medications that alter the perception of chest pain include analgesics (narcotic, nonnarcotic), anxiolytics, and hypnotics. As one may anticipate, the influence of medications and comorbid illnesses is most profound in the elderly.

Psychosocial factors exert an important influence on pain perception. Individuals in higher social strata typically have a broader spectrum of coping mechanisms at their disposal. The use of problem-

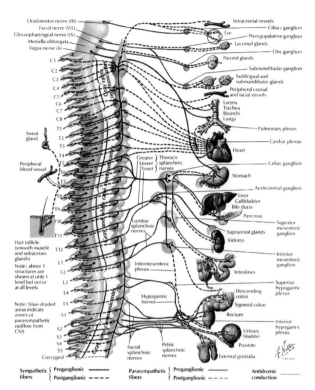

Figure 2-2. The autonomic nervous system consists of afferent components, integrating systems, and effector pathways. The perception of pain from visceral organs is poorly localized because of specialized functions that have teleologically replaced basic sensory receptors. (Copyright 1989. Novartis. Reprinted with permission from the Atlas of Human Anatomy, illustrated by Frank H. Netter, M.D. All rights reserved.)

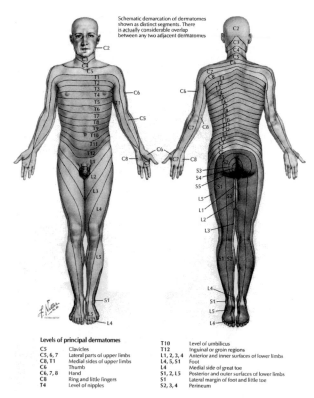

Schematic demarcation of dermatomes shown as distinct segments. There is actually considerable overlap between any two adjacent dermatomes

Levels of principal dermatomes

C5	Clavicles	T10	Level of umbilicus
C5, 6, 7	Lateral parts of upper limbs	T12	Inguinal or groin regions
C8, T1	Medial sides of upper limbs	L1, 2, 3, 4	Anterior and inner surfaces of lower limbs
C6	Thumb	L4, 5, S1	Foot
C6, 7, 8	Hand	L4	Medial side of great toe
C8	Ring and little fingers	S1, 2, L5	Posterior and outer surfaces of lower limbs
T4	Level of nipples	S1	Lateral margin of foot and little toe
		S2, 3, 4	Perineum

Figure 2-3. The cutaneous distribution of sensory perception is represented schematically by demarcated regions, or dermatomes. Despite the apparently well-defined areas, there is considerable overlap between adjacent dermatomes. (Copyright 1989. Novartis. Reprinted with permission from the Atlas of Human Anatomy, illustrated by Frank H. Netter, M.D. All rights reserved.)

oriented coping styles reduces pain perception. In contrast, depression increases pain awareness. This is a particularly important contributor to chronic pain syndromes.

Because women delay in seeking evaluation for chest pain symptoms compared with men, many have speculated that differing pain thresholds are operational. There is no clear evidence that pain thresholds differ between men and women; however, a women's perception of pain and the psychosocial response that follows is unique. Age, life experiences, and concomitant social conditions also have a significant influence and, in general, tend to attenuate pain itself and/or the response to pain. The same is true of varying cultures where "expression" may either be condoned or condemned.

DYNAMICS OF PAIN

There are four cutaneous senses: *touch-pressure, cold, warmth,* and *pain.* The sensory organs for pain are the naked nerve endings found in a majority of bodily tissues. Pain senses are transmitted to the central nervous system by small myelinated (A) fibers and unmyelinated (C) fibers. The latter conduct at a slower rate. The existence of separate pathways explains the sharp nature of most sudden-onset painful sensations followed by a persistence that is characteristically less intense.

The autonomic nervous system, like the skin, joints, and muscles (somatic sensory organs), has afferent components, integrating stations, and effector pathways. Pain from visceral structures is poorly localized, unpleasant, associated with nausea and other autonomic symptoms, and often radiates or is "referred" to other areas. The poor localization of visceral pain is due to the relative paucity of pain receptors that, in essence, have been telelogically replaced by specialized nerve functions—osmoreceptors, baroreceptors, and chemoreceptors. However, visceral pain, like somatic pain, can initiate reflex contraction of nearby skeletal muscle. The spasm of surrounding muscles (for example, the rigidity of abdominal muscles in the setting of a perforated viscus) may protect the involved structures from further trauma.[2,3]

ASSESSMENT OF PAIN

No objective tests can fully assess the severity of pain or even its presence. Therefore, the physician must accept the patient's account, taking into consideration his or her age, cultural background, environment, and psychologic circumstances known to influence the reaction to pain.

A thorough history, general physical examination, and careful neurologic examination are imperative in any patient complaining of pain. Inquiry should be made concerning (1) the temporal pattern of pain, (2) its distribution, (3) exacerbating factors, and (4) relieving factors.

A careful psychiatric history, searching particularly for signs and symptoms of depression, should be elicited from all patients. The distinction between "pain" and "suffering" should be made by both the physician and the patient.

A general physical examination must be performed early in the evaluation of patients with pain. Both the physical and the laboratory examinations should begin with the assumption that the site of pathologic change is at the site of pain. The painful areas should be examined for swelling and redness as well as for any obvious deformity. The areas reported as painful should be palpated, the temperature estimated, and points of tenderness sought. (If the site of pain is in a soft tissue, bone, or joint, it should be tender to palpation as well as spontaneously painful.) Finally, laboratory examinations and other diagnostic tests should be obtained as a means to confirm the clinician's suspicions.

THE ART OF VISUALIZATION

Throughout time clinicians have utilized the art of visualization toward developing physical diagnosis skills in favor of rote memorization and its inherent limitations. In general terms, one begins the artful journey before words are outwardly spoken by inwardly asking the question, How does the patient look? Even the inexperienced clinician with an untrained eye can make an initial observation of "wellness" or "unwellness" that should immediately illicit a feeling of concern. The experienced clinician recognizes that the *initial impression* is a vital component of patient assessment that guides the evaluation to follow; but perhaps of greatest importance, the astute clinician never underestimates the signs, symptoms, and feelings of "unwellness" that prompts an individual to seek medical attention and, in essence, ask for help.

With each step in the evaluation process, the clinician must remain "open-minded" and unbiased, considering the possible diagnosis carefully. In the final analysis, a diagnosis should never be made prematurely (before all the necessary information is gathered and evaluated).

REFERENCES

1. Besson J-M. The neurobiology of pain. Lancet 1999;353:1610–1615.
2. Strunin L (ed). Postgraduate educational issue: inflammatory and neurogenic pain: new molecules, new mechanisms. Br J Anaesthesiol 1995; 75:123–255.
3. Lipkowski AW, Carr DB. Neuropeptides: peptide and nonpeptide analogs. In B Gutte (ed), Peptides: Synthesis, Structures, and Applications. New York: Academic Press, 1995.

PART TWO

Assessment of Chest Pain

Anatomic Considerations

The chest or, more anatomically speaking, the thoracic cavity is bounded posteriorly by the vertebral column and ribs, laterally by the ribs alone, anteriorly by the ribs and sternum, and superiorly by an imaginary plane at the level of the first ribs.[1]

The thoracic cavity is frequently subdivided into three portions:

1. Left pleural cavity
2. Right pleural cavity
3. Mediastinum

The mediastinum itself is divided into *superior* and *inferior* portions, with the latter anatomically subdivided into anterior, middle, and posterior compartments (Figure 3-1).

The *superior mediastinum* contains the following structures: thymus, superior vena cava, bracheocephalic vein, aorta and its major branches, pulmonary trunk, and trachea and esophagus.

The *anterior* chamber of the *inferior mediastinum* contains predominantly fat and connective tissue; while the *middle* chamber houses the heart, pericardium, and origins of the great vessels. The *posterior* mediastinum includes the descending aorta, esophagus, vagus nerve, hemiazygous vein, accessory hemiazygous vein, thoracic duct, and sympathetic chains.

The anatomic relationships between structures found within the thoracic cavity are vital for understanding chest pain, as are the relationships between the thoracic and abdominal cavities (Figure 3-2).

NORMAL CORONARY ANATOMY

Blood and essential substrates are carried to the myocardium through the major epicardial coronary arteries, their branches, intramural and subendocardial extensions (microcirculation), and the collateral circulation.

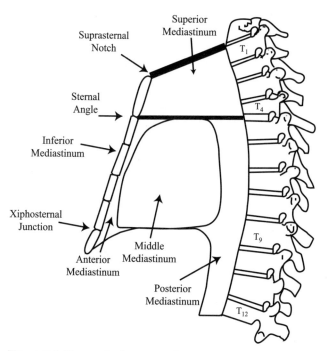

Figure 3-1. The mediastinum contains two distinct sections: the superior mediastinum and the inferior mediastinum. The inferior mediastinum is further subdivided anatomically into the anterior, middle, and posterior compartments.

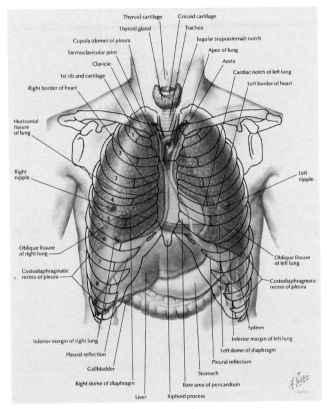

Figure 3-2. The thoracic cavity contains the lungs, heart, and great vessels. Its anatomic relationship with the abdominal cavity is vital to understanding the comprehensive evaluation of chest pain. (Copyright 1989. Novartis. Reprinted with permission from the Atlas of Human Anatomy, illustrated by Frank H. Netter, M.D. All rights reserved.)

Right Coronary Artery

The right coronary artery (RCA), typically 2.5 to 3.0 mm in diameter, originates within the right coronary sinus of Valsalva (Figure 3-3). It extends between the right atrium and right ventricle in the atrioventricular groove. In approximately 80% of individuals, the RCA reaches the crux cordis and gives rise to posterior descending, atrioventricular node (AV) and left ventricular branches.

The branches of the RCA beginning proximally near the vessel's origin include:

- Conus branch

- SA nodal branch

- Right atrial branch

- Right ventricular marginal branches

- Posterolateral branch

- AV nodal branch

- Posterior descending branch

- Septal branch

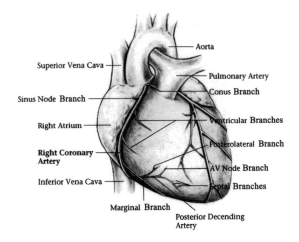

Figure 3-3. Anatomy of the right coronary artery.

LEFT CORONARY ARTERY

The left coronary artery originates in the left coronary sinus of the Valsalva. The ostium typically is located at the level of the aortic ring, up to 1.0 cm higher than the ostium of the RCA (Figure 3-4). The left main coronary artery, which may be up to 4.5 mm in diameter, divides into two major

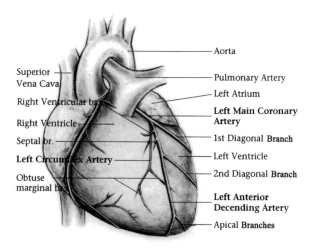

Aorta

Pulmonary Artery

Left Atrium

Left Main Coronary Artery

1st Diagonal Branch

Left Ventricle

2nd Diagonal Branch

Left Anterior Decending Artery

Apical Branches

Superior Vena Cava

Right Ventricular br.

Right Ventricle

Septal br.

Left Circumflex Artery

Obtuse marginal br.

Figure 3-4. Anatomy of the left coronary artery, including the left main, left anterior descending, and left circumflex coronary arteries.

branches: the left anterior descending (LAD) coronary artery and the left circumflex coronary artery. Rarely, these vessels may arise from separate ostia located within the left coronary sinus.

The branches of the LAD beginning proximally are as follows:

- Diagonal branch

- Septal branch

- Right ventricular branch

- Apical branch

The *left circumflex coronary artery* commonly takes off at a sharp angle from the left main coronary artery and courses posteriorly in the AV groove toward the crux cordis. In 80% of individuals, the left circumflex artery does not reach the posterior interventricular sulcus. When it does, however, the left circumflex artery gives rise to a posterior descending branch that is the sole source of blood supply to the posterior interventricular septum and the AV node. In 40% of individuals, the left circumflex artery provides a branch to the sinus node.

The longest and most consistent branches of the left circumflex artery are those to the acute margin of the heart: the obtuse marginal branches.

The coronary circulation has been divided anatomically into dominant and nondominant, depending on which blood vessel reaches and crosses the crux cordis of the heart. In this instance the posterior descending artery and often the AV nodal artery originate from the dominant vessel. Accordingly, the RCA is considered the *dominant* vessel in approximately 80% of individuals. However, the left coronary artery system provides blood flow to the largest area of myocardium and therefore is the *predominant* artery in most individuals.

CORONARY ARTERY ANOMALIES

For oxygen to be delivered to metabolically active myocardial cells, coronary arterial blood flow must be adequate. Clearly, normal coronary arterial blood flow requires normal coronary artery anatomy (epicardial and microvascular). In some cases, anatomic variations (anomalies) preclude normal delivery of essential substrate, compromising myocardial function.

Coronary Ostial Abnormalities

The coronary ostium can be abnormal with respect to its intrinsic anatomy (proper aortic sinus origin), size (ostial hyperplasia, fibrous endoproliferation, atresia), or orientation (tangential orientation, intussusception).

Ectopic Coronary Artery Origination

Coronary arteries can originate from the pulmonary trunk. There also may be anomalous origin from an atypical site: a noncoronary cusp, the aortic wall above the coronary sinus, or the descending aorta.

The right coronary artery, left main coronary artery, left anterior descending coronary artery, or left circumflex coronary artery can have an anomalous origin. The course taken can be posterior to the aorta, between the aorta and pulmonary trunk, within the ventricular septum, or anterior to the pulmonary infundibulum. Other arteries can have ectopic origins, arising from an extracardiac vessel (subclavin artery, internal thoracic artery, brachiocephalic artery, carotid artery) or from a heart chamber (left ventricle, right ventricle).

Abnormal Connections

Abnormal connections between a coronary artery and an adjacent vascular structure tend to enlarge with time because of the persistence of a pressure gradient. Examples are a coronary-cameral fistula (right ventricle, left ventricle, right atrium, left atrium), coronary arteriovenous fistula, and coronary to extracardiac artery or vein (coronary-pulmonary, coronary-bronchial, coronary-caval) fistula.

Intramural Coursing (Muscular Bridge)

The main coronary arteries and their branches course on the epicardial surface of the heart. Occasionally, the vessels take a subepicardial course. On rare occasions, the coronary arteries become intracavitary or subendocardial. An exception is the LAD coronary artery, which in its midportion takes a subepicardial course in nearly 50% of individuals (which therefore is considered a normal anatomic variant).

Coronary Artery Size

The diameter of a coronary artery can be too small (hypoplastic) or too large (ectatic). Either may be a congenital or acquired abnormality. Coronary artery ectasia with aneurysm formation is seen with coronary arteritis and atherosclerosis as well as following trauma.

REFERENCES

1. Craft RC. Textbook of Human Anatomy. New York: John Wiley and Sons, 1966.

Physiologic Considerations

As a general rule, organs and tissues with adequate blood supply and substrate for physiologic cellular metabolism function normally. Disruption of this fundamental homeostatic balance often leads to dysfunction, tissue damage, and depending on the involved organ, pain.

The heart perhaps is the most sensitive organ to *shifts* in supply and demand. The major determinants of myocardial oxygenation consumption (demand) are wall tension (pressure X volume), inotropic state (contractility), heart rate, and myocardial mass.[1,2]

OXYGEN-CARRYING CAPACITY
OF BLOOD

The complex structural and functional properties of hemoglobin allow erythrocytes to bind, transport, and release oxygen with great efficiency. The interior of a normal erythrocyte contains nearly 300 million molecules of hemoglobin. Each molecule is a tetramer composed of polypeptide chains, to which four heme moieties are bound. Hemoglobins found in normal adults include hemoglobin A (97% total), hemoglobin A_2 (2%), and hemoglobin F (1%).

The unique physiologic role of hemoglobin in tissue metabolism is fostered by the sigmoidal shape of its oxygen-binding curve. In reality, hemoglobin has a relatively low oxygen affinity. With decreasing pH and increasing 2,3-diphosphoglyceric acid (DPG) concentrations or temperature, a further decrease in hemoglobin's affinity for oxygen occurs, causing more oxygen to be released at the tissue level for a given PO_2.

Hemoglobin's ability to function as an oxygen transporter depends on its ability to bind oxygen and release it at the tissue level. An increased affinity for oxygen reduces tissue PO_2 and may compromise cellular function and viability. A decreased affinity may significantly affect oxygen transport. Genetic and acquired abnormalities of hemoglobin do occur. Although a majority of individuals are asymptomatic, anemia (in patients with decreased oxygen affinity) and erythrocytosis (in patients with increased oxygen affinity) may be seen.

CORONARY BLOOD FLOW

With increasing myocardial demands, oxygen consumption increases three- to fourfold. Since myocardial oxygen extraction cannot increase substantially, coronary blood flow must increase to meet demands placed on the heart.[3,4]

The factors known to influence coronary blood flow include:

- Duration of diastole

- Perfusion pressure gradient (aortic-left ventricular end-diastolic pressure difference)

- Autoregulation

- Neurohumoral tone

- Metabolic state

REFERENCES

1. Epstein SE, Talbot TL. Dynamic coronary tone in precipitation, exacerbation and relief of angina pectoris. Am J Cardiol 1981;48:797–803.
2. Braunwald E, Sobel BE. Coronary blood flow and myocardial ischemia. In E Braunwald (ed), Heart Disease (4th ed). Philadelphia: WB Saunders, 1992;1161–1165.
3. Factor SM, Kirk ES. Pathophysiology of myocardial ischemia. In JW Hurst, RB Logue, CE Rackley, et al. (eds), The Heart (6th ed). New York: McGraw-Hill, 1986;856–860.
4. Rouleau J, Boerboom LE, Surjadhana A, et al. The role of autoregulation and tissue diastolic pressures in the transmural distribution of left ventricular blood flow in anesthetized dogs. Circ Res 1979;45:804–815.

Differential Diagnosis

Chest pain is a particularly common complaint among patients undergoing evaluation in Urgent Care Clinics and Emergency Departments. It can represent a cardiac, vascular, gastrointestinal, pulmonary, musculoskeletal, psychologic, neurologic, or dermatologic disorder. Chest pain accounts for an estimated 2–4% of all Emergency Department visits in the United States and nearly 2 million Americans are admitted to Intensive Care Units yearly with suspected acute myocardial ischemia (Figure 5-1 and Table 5-1).

It is common in clinical practice to err on the conservative or safe side when evaluating patients with chest pain and suspected myocardial ischemia.

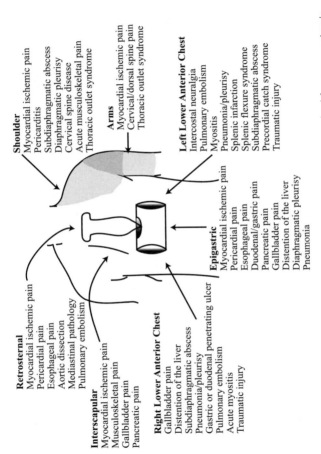

Shoulder
Myocardial ischemic pain
Pericarditis
Subdiaphragmatic abscess
Diaphragmatic pleurisy
Cervical spine disease
Acute musculoskeletal pain
Thoracic outlet syndrome

Arms
Myocardial ischemic pain
Cervical/dorsal spine pain
Thoracic outlet syndrome

Left Lower Anterior Chest
Intercostal neuralgia
Pulmonary embolism
Myositis
Pneumonia/pleurisy
Splenic infarction
Splenic flexure syndrome
Subdiaphragmatic abscess
Precordial catch syndrome
Traumatic injury

Retrosternal
Myocardial ischemic pain
Pericardial pain
Esophageal pain
Aortic dissection
Mediastinal pathology
Pulmonary embolism

Interscapular
Myocardial ischemic pain
Musculoskeletal pain
Gallbladder pain
Pancreatic pain

Right Lower Anterior Chest
Gallbladder pain
Distention of the liver
Subdiaphragmatic abscess
Pneumonia/pleurisy
Gastric or duodenal penetrating ulcer
Pulmonary embolism
Acute myositis
Traumatic injury

Epigastric
Myocardial ischemic pain
Pericardial pain
Esophageal pain
Duodenal/gastric pain
Pancreatic pain
Gallbladder pain
Distention of the liver
Diaphragmatic pleurisy
Pneumonia

Figure 5-1. The differential diagnosis of chest pain is best approached from an anatomic perspective. (Adapted with permission from AJ Miller. Diagnosis of Chest Pain. New York: Raven Press, 1988;175.)

Failure to recognize unstable angina, acute myocardial infarction, and other life-threatening causes of chest pain could have serious consequences for the patient, family members, medical team, and the institution. In addition, recent advances in therapies that achieve myocardial salvage (coronary fibrinolysis, primary coronary angioplasty) provide a unique opportunity to affect the clinical outcome when a correct diagnosis is made expeditiously.

Unfortunately, there is considerable overlap in the signs and symptoms of myocardial ischemia and other cardiac and noncardiac causes of chest pain.[1]

Table 5-1. Differential diagnosis of chest pain

Cardiac
  Ischemic
    Atherosclerotic
    Coronary spasm
    Systemic hypertension
    Pulmonary hypertension
    Aortic stenosis
    Aortic insufficiency
    Hypertrophic cardiomy-
      opathy
    Severe anemia
    Severe hypoxia
    Polycythemia
    Nonatherosclerotic epi-
      dial disease
  Nonischemic
    Aortic dissection
    Aortic aneurysm
    Pericarditis
    Mitral valve prolapse
    Myocarditis
    Cardiomyopathy
Noncardiac
  Pulmonary
    Pulmonary embolism
    Pneumothorax
    Pneumonia
    Pleuritis
    Bronchospasm
    Pulmonary hypertension
    Tracheitis and tracheo-
      bronchitis

    Intrathoracic tumor
Gastrointestinal
  Motility disorders
    Nutcracker esophagus
    Diffuse esophageal
      spasm
    Nonspecific motility
      disorder
    Achalasia
  Gastroesophageal reflux
  Esophageal rupture
    (Boerhaave's syn-
      drome)
  Esophageal tear (Mallory-
    Weiss syndrome)
  Esophagitis
    Candida
    Herpes
    Irradiation induced
  Esophageal foreign body
  Peptic ulcer disease
  Pancreatitis
  Biliary disease (cholecys-
    titis or biliary colic)
  Splenic infarction
  Gaseous bowel disten-
    tion
Neuromusculoskeletal
  Thoracic outlet syndrome
    Anterior scalene hyper-
      trophy
    Cervical rib

Table 5-1. *continued*

Cervical disk disease
Costochondritis/Tietze's syndrome
Chest wall trauma/rib fracture
Malignancy
Herpes zoster
Precordial catch syndrome
Sternal wire nerve entrapment
Xiphodynia
Slipping rib syndrome
Ostalgia due to neoplasm, inflammation, or infarction
Sternal marrow pain (acute leukemia)
Intercostal neuritis
Reflex autonomic dysfunction

Psychiatric
 Depression
 Anxiety
 Panic attacks
 Malingering
Other
 Cocaine
 Lymphoma
 Diabetes
 Uremia
 Renal stones
 Superficial thrombophlebitis (Mondor's syndrome)
 Mediastinitis
 Mediastinal emphysema
 Mediastinal neoplasms

REFERENCES

1. Rutledge JC, Amsterdam EA. Differential diagnosis and clinical approach to the patient with acute chest pain. Cardiol clin 1984;2:257–268.

CHAPTER SIX

Cardiac Chest Pain

Chest pain is part of the symptom complex for most patients with acute ischemic heart disease. The pain of *angina pectoris* has a diverse presentation. Some episodes of myocardial ischemia or infarction may occur without chest pain, but produce "anginal equivalents," including profound weakness, diaphoresis, nausea, malaise, dyspnea, and localized discomfort in areas more commonly affected by radiating pain (epigastrium, arms, back). The incidence of atypical symptoms associated with myocardial ischemia increases with older age, diabetes, prior stroke, spinal cord disease, and following either coronary artery bypass surgery or cardiac transplantation. Up to 15% of myocardial infarctions are either clinically silent or masked by coexisting conditions (e.g., following trauma or major surgery).

Ischemic chest pain is not synonymous with chest pain due to atherosclerosis. In addition to atherosclerotic epicardial coronary artery disease, a variety of cardiac abnormalities can produce similar symptoms (Table 6-1).

The classic description of ischemic chest pain was offered by William Heberden over two centuries ago: "But there is a disorder of the breast marked with strong and peculiar symptoms, considerable for the kind of danger belonging to it, and not extremely rare. The seat of it, and the sense of strangling and anxiety with which it is attended, may make it not improperly called angina pectoris."[1]

PATIENT HISTORY

The clinician should meticulously investigate the patient's symptoms through a careful and orderly history (Table 6-2).

Location/Radiation

Ischemic pain typically is located in the lower substernal area. It may radiate to one or both arms, the shoulders, anterior neck, lower jaw, and less often, the teeth, wrists, and back. The extreme limits of radiation are from the occiput to the epigastrium.

Quality

Ischemic cardiac pain typically is a deep visceral sensation and therefore frequently is described as choking, constricting, heavy, squeezing, suffocating, strangling, pressure, burning, viselike, bandlike, and discomfort, not pain, "like someone standing on my chest." The intensity ranges from mild to crushing. Rarely is ischemic chest pain described as well localized, sharp, stabbing, knifelike, or tearing in quality. Associated symptoms include diaphoresis, hiccoughing, dyspnea, and nausea.

The patient's description of discomfort may be influenced by socioeconomic, educational, cultural, and historical variables and by emotional state.

Duration

In most instances, ischemic chest pain lasts 2–20 minutes. Pain lasting greater than 30 minutes should raise the suspicion of acute MI (myocardial infarction) or a nonischemic etiology.

Table 6-1. Nonatherosclerotic epicardial coronary diseases

Arteritis
  Syphilis
  Tuberculosis
  Takayasu's disease
  Giant cell
  Kawasaki disease
  Polyarteritis nodosa
Collagen vascular
  Rheumatoid arthritis
  Systemic lupus erythemato-
    sus
  Systemic sclerosis
Coronary mural thickening
  Mucopolysaccharidosis
    (Hunter's syndrome)
  Homocysteinuria
  Fabry's disease
  Amyloidosis
  Juvenile intimal sclerosis
  Pseudoxanthoma elasticum
External compression
  Tumor
  Amyloidosis
  Mural thrombosis (left
    ventricular)
  Iatrogenic
  Infectious endocarditis
  Marantic endocarditis
  Thromboembolism
  Fibromyxoma of aortic
    valve
  Atrial myxoma

Coronary spasm
  Prinzmetal's angina
  Cocaine
  Industrial nitroglycerin
    withdrawal
Coronary ostial occlusion
  Takayasu's disease
  Syphilis
  Aortic Starr-Edward's
    prosthetic valve
  Congenital supravalvular
    aortic stenosis
Coronary artery anomalies
  Coronary atrioventricular
    fistula
  Anomalous left coronary
    artery from pulmonary
    trunk
Trauma
  Coronary artery lacera-
    tion
  Sinus of Valsalva aneurysm
Coronary aneurysms
  Congenital
  Atherosclerotic
  Traumatic
Coronary embolism
  Cardiomyopathy
  Mitral stenosis
Coronary artery thrombo-
    sis
  Myocardial contusion

Table 6-1. *continued*

Coronary artery dissection
Electrical, thermal, or radia-
    tion trauma
Arterial dissection
    Aortic dissection
    Spontaneous coronary dis-
        section

**Table 6-2. Key determinants for evaluating patients
with chest pain**

*The clinician should determine the following
characteristics:*

- Location
- Radiation
- Character
- Precipitants
- Alleviants
- Duration
- Frequency
- Pattern
- Associated symptoms

Precipitants and Alleviants

Ischemic chest pain often is precipitated by exertion and can be provoked by emotional stress, a large meal, the supine position (angina decubitus), sexual intercourse, cold weather, and use of the upper extremities. The intensity of effort necessary to incite angina frequently varies from day-to-day and throughout a given day; often, the threshold is lower in the morning, after large meals, during cold weather, and with emotional upset. It may be relieved by rest within 2–10 minutes, nitrates within 2–5 minutes, standing, carotid sinus massage, oxygen, or beta-blockade.

Chest pain associated with MI frequently is more severe and radiates more widely. Although it may be, it typically is not triggered by exertion or emotional stress, is not relieved by rest, and often is associated with diaphoresis, nausea, fatigue, vomiting, dyspnea, and a sense of "impending doom."

The heart and its major supporting structure (the pericardium) are a common source of chest pain. Anatomically and physiologically cardiac chest pain is frequently divided into *ischemic* and *nonischemic* pain.

ISCHEMIC PAIN

Scope of the Problem

Ischemic chest pain is common and represents a major public health challenge. The prevalence has been difficult to establish but the American Heart Association has estimated that over 6 million Americans have ischemic chest pain and an equal number have silent coronary artery disease.

Ischemic chest pain is important not only because of its prevalence but also because of the underlying process that it most often represents—atherosclerotic coronary artery disease. Ischemic heart disease is the leading cause of death in the United States, responsible for 1 of every 4.8 deaths. The financial burden is enormous with $15 billion in hospitalization costs alone each year.

Disorders of Myocardial Oxygen Supply

Coronary Atherosclerosis

In the vast majority of patients with documented myocardial ischemia or infarction, coronary atherosclerosis is the underlying pathologic process. Clinical manifestations of coronary atherosclerosis follow chronic as well as acute reductions in epicardial coronary arterial blood flow and myocardial perfusion. Atherosclerotic narrowing of the epicardial coronary vessels, while diffuse in nature, can be accelerated locally with a propensity toward more proximally positioned segments and at branch points.

A large body of evidence suggests the conversion from stable to unstable angina is heralded by plaque disruption (erosion, rupture, fissuring), which exposes the atherosclerotic matrix and subendothelium to circulating blood products (platelets and coagulation factors).

The precise cause of plaque disruption is unknown; however, most rupture events occur within soft plaques that are rich in cholesterol, cholesterol esters, macrophages, and activated lympocytes. The site of rupture typically is at the plaques "shoulder" region where the fibrous cap and adjacent uninvolved vascular layer join. Possible inciting mechanisms leading to plaque rupture are shearing forces caused by the stenosis itself, coronary vasospasm, and twisting (torquing) of the coronary artery during ventricular systolic in the cardiac cycle. In addition, macrophages that degrade the plaques internal supporting framework through the release of matrix metaloproteinases contribute substantially.

Platelets attracted to a region of vascular injury and plaque disruption facilitate ischemic episodes through a variety of mechanisms. Their clinical importance is underscored by the finding of platelet aggregates within the microvasculature among patients with unstable angina experiencing cardiac death. Platelets episodically occlude or markedly reduce coronary flow through locally stenotic segments by aggregation.

Coronary Vasospasm

A proportionately large number of ischemic episodes are the result of increased myocardial oxygen demand; however, a primary reduction in coronary blood flow (from thrombotic occlusion and/or vasospasm) also is common. Interest in coronary vasospasm as a precipitant of myocardial ischemia originated within the observed occurrence of angina (or other features of myocardial ischemia) in patients with coronary atherosclerosis and no overt evidence of increased oxygen demand.

Coronary vasospasm most often occurs at sites of atherosclerosis and accompanying endothelial cell dysfunction overlying an atherosclerotic plaque (Figure 6-1). Normal coronary arteries dilate in response to mental stress and physical exercise, whereas diseased vessels contract. Although the precise cause of altered vasomotion in atherosclerotic vessels is not clear, a quantitative defect in the elaboration of nitric oxide has been postulated.[2]

While the vast majority of patients exhibiting myocardial ischemia and infarction have underlying coronary atherosclerosis, nonatherosclerotic coronary disease also should be considered as a possible etiology, particularly in patients without identifiable risk factors.

Congenital Abnormalities

Isolated congenital anomalies of the coronary arteries are identified in less than 1% of adults undergoing coronary angiography. The most common abnormality is characterized by origination of the left circumflex artery from the right coronary sinus of Valsalva or as a branch of the right coronary artery. Origin of the left coronary artery from the pulmonary artery (Bland-White-Garland syndrome) is rare among adults but is associated with increased incidence of myocardial ischemia and sudden cardiac death.

Aberrant origination of the left or right coronary arteries from the "wrong" sinus of Valsalva is rare but can be of clinical significance. Sudden car-

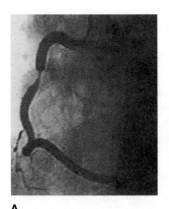 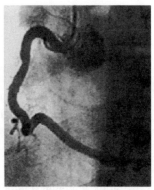

A

B

Figure 6-1. Selective right coronary angiogram in a patient with clinical and electrocardiographic signs of acute myocardial infarction. (A) A high-grade stenosis is visualized in the vessel's mid-portion. (B) The vessel lumen is more normal in appearance following intracoronary administration of nitroglycerin. (Reprinted with permission from CD Kimmelstiel, CA Clyne, RC Becker. Mechanisms of acute myocardial ischemia and infarction. In RS Irwin, FB Cerra, JM Rippe [eds], Irwin and Rippe's Intensive Care Medicine [4th ed]. Philadelphia: Lippincott–Raven, 1999;1:545.)

diac death can occur after strenuous physical exercise and among patients in whom the aberrant vessel courses *between* the aorta and pulmonary artery. The ostium of the vessel frequently is underdeveloped and slitlike. In addition, its anatomic course frequently takes an acute angle effecting functional coronary internal dimensions.

Coronary arteriovenous (AV) fistulas can cause myocardial ischemia through a "steal phenomenon," where left-to-right shunting deprives the myocardium of oxygenated blood. Most AV fistulas are congenital, but acquired forms can develop following trauma or coronary bypass grafting.[3]

Trauma

Penetrating and blunt trauma can cause myocardial ischemia and infarction. Penetrating trauma (e.g., stabbing or gunshot wound) can cause coronary lacerations, although the most common clinical presentation in this setting is pericardial tamponade. Blunt trauma can cause myocardial necrosis (even in the absence of preexisting atherosclerotic disease).

Embolism

Embolism to an epicardial coronary artery can cause myocardial ischemia or infarction. The LAD is the vessel most commonly involved. Potential sources of emboli include left ventricular mural thrombus, endocarditis (either native or prosthetic valve), malignancy (primary, metastatic), air emboli during cardiac surgery or cardiac catheterization, paradoxical embolization (venous to arterial system) across a patent foramen ovale, ventricular septal defect, and/or atrial septal defect.[4]

Dissection

Coronary arterial dissection provokes myocardial ischemia and infarction when the vessel's intima separates from the media and the resultant "flap" obstructs blood flow through the vessel's lumen. Obstructive dissections occur most commonly as a complication of percutaneous coronary interventions and rarely following of diagnostic angiography. An ascending aortic dissection may propagate in a retrograde fashion to involve the coronary ostia. Spontaneous coronary artery dissection has been described, with a majority occurring during pregnancy or shortly after delivery. Spontaneous dissection also occurs in the presence of advanced atherosclerosis. Most cases involve the LAD.

Anemia

A sudden decrease in circulating blood volume can reduce myocardial perfusion and, as a result, precipitate myocardial ischemia. Chronic, severe anemia (hematocrit <22%) can produce a high output state, increasing myocardial oxygen demand.

Hypotension

Myocardial perfusion is determined, in large part, by systemic perfusion pressure. Therefore, systemic hypotension, if severe and prolonged, can precipitate myocardial ischemia. The maintenance of mean arterial pressure is particularly important among patients with coexisting coronary artery disease in whom coronary flow is compromised at baseline even under ideal hemodynamic circumstances.

Disorders of Myocardial Oxygen Demand

Aortic Stenosis

Angina pectoris is a common clinical manifestation of aortic stenosis. Even in the absence of coronary disease, myocardial oxygen demand can exceed supply due to myocardial hypertrophy, prolongation of the systolic ejection period, and elevated left ventricular and diastolic pressure. In addition, increased left ventricular systolic pressure can externally compress intramyocardial coronary vessels, disrupting flow to the subendocardium.

Aortic Insufficiency

Myocardial ischemia can develop among patients with aortic insufficiency and left ventricular dilation. An increased myocardial oxygen demand coupled with diminished systemic diastolic pressure, a hallmark of chronic aortic insufficiency, reduces coronary perfusion.

Hypertensive Heart Disease

Long-standing, poorly controlled hypertension is associated with the development of left ventricular hypertrophy and atherosclerotic coronary artery disease. Left ventricular hypertrophy, even in the absence of coexisting coronary disease, can cause myocardial ischemia as a consequence of increased myocardial mass (and oxygen demand) combined with diminished perfusion pressure, relating to elevated left ventricular end-diastolic pressure.

Hypertrophic Cardiomyopathy

In hypertrophic obstructive cardiomyopathy, a significant increase in myocardial mass may compromise perfusion. Myocardial oxygen demand may be particularly high in patients with left ventricular outflow tract gradients.

High-Output States

In high-output states such as hyperthyroidism, ischemic chest pain is most likely to occur in patients with underlying coronary artery disease in whom elevated myocardial oxygen demand is precipitated by increased contractility and heart rate. Coronary arterial spasm also has been reported in patients with hyperthyroidism.

Dilated Cardiomyopathy

The dilated ventricular has increased oxygen demands, particularly in the setting of decompensated heart failure where elevated left ventricular end-diastolic pressure compromises myocardial perfusion.

NONISCHEMIC CARDIAC PAIN

Abnormal Cardiac Sensitivity

Right ventricle catheter manipulation, right atrial pacing, and intracoronary contrast injection is perceived as chest pain more often in patients with chest pain syndromes and normal coronary arteries than in those with angiographically significant coronary disease. These observations suggest that cardiac hypersensitivity may be either causally related or contributory in some patients with chest pain. Alternatively, cardiac hypersensitivity may be a marker of generalized visceral hypersensitivity.

Mitral Valve Prolapse

A chest pain syndrome has been described in patients with mitral valve prolapse. While symptoms may be suggestive of angina pectoris, in many cases they are atypical (well localized to the precordium) and occur sporadically with or without exertion. Rest pain is reported more often and tends to vary in duration from seconds to hours. The location, response to nitrates, and site(s) of radiation also vary from one episode to the next. Palpitations, lightheadedness, syncope, chronic fatigue, anxiety, depression, and hyperventilation are common accompanying symptoms.

The pathophysiology of chest pain among patients with mitral valve prolapse has not been fully elucidated; however, tension on the chordae tendineae and papillary muscle apparatus produced by the tethered and "billowing" valve may cause focal ischemia. This mechanism also may help explain the rare but reported association between mitral valve prolapse and sudden cardiac death. In a majority of patients, however, the chest pain is not ischemic in nature.

Acute Pericarditis

The symptoms associated with pericarditis typically are sharp, stabbing, parasternal chest pain that is pleuritic in nature, radiating to the left trapezius ridge. It can be relieved by sitting forward and aggravated by assuming the prone position, swallowing, coughing, or twisting. The pain, which can be reproduced with deep palpation, often lasts for hours and sometimes mimics angina, particularly when it occurs in the post-MI setting.

Patients with pericarditis often are young and have few risk factors for atherosclerosis coronary artery disease. Pericarditis has many underlying causes, including recent MI (<7 days), prior MI (30–42 days—Dressler's syndrome), aortic dissection, viral syndrome, trauma uremia, tuberculosis, and collagen vascular diseases.

REFERENCES

1. Heberden W. Commentaries on the history and cure of diseases. In FA Willius, TE Keys (eds), Classics of Cardiology. New York: Henry Schuman, Dover Publications, 1941;I:221.
2. Maseri A, Chierchia S, Kaski JC. Mixed angina pectoris. Am J Cardiol 1985;56:30E–33E.

3. Levin DC, Fellows KE, Abrams HL. Hemodynamically significant primary anomalies of the coronary arteries: Angiographic aspects. Circulation 1978;58:25–34.
4. Nachman RL, Silverstein R. Hypercoagulable states. Ann Intern Med 1993;119:819–827.

Noncardiac Chest Pain

PULMONARY CAUSES OF CHEST PAIN

Pulmonary Hypertension

The discomfort experienced by patients with pulmonary hypertension has qualities that are reminiscent of typical angina. This is because, in some cases, the symptoms may be caused by right ventricular ischemia (right heart strain) or dilation of the pulmonary arteries.[1] Potential causes of pulmonary hypertension include massive pulmonary embolism, primary pulmonary hypertension, severe chronic obstructive lung disease, mitral stenosis, and severe long-standing left ventricular failure. The diagnostic challenge is created by the high incidence of concomitant coronary disease; however, a careful physical examination and interpretation of an ECG, chest X ray, and other diagnostic tests (perfusion imaging, echocardiogram) provide the necessary means to discriminate between cardiac and pulmonary pathology. Severe pulmonic stenosis can cause chest pain, presumably because of right ventricular subendocardial ischemia.

Pleuritis

Inflammation or distention of the pleura causes chest pain that is worsened by deep inspiration and coughing. Movement and palpation have less of an effect. A physical examination may reveal fever, pleural friction rub, pleural effusion(s), and pulmonary consolidation. Pleural inflammation can have many causes. Pleurodynia, a self-limited disease caused by coxsackie B infection, causes pleuritic chest pain. Usually, a viral prodrome precedes the development of chest discomfort by 7–10 days.

Pneumonia

When infectious pneumonia extends from the lung parenchyma to the pleural surface, pleuritic chest pain may occur. The accompanying fever, cough, dyspnea, sputum production, elevated white blood cell count, and radiographic findings provide support for the diagnosis. Bronchospasm and cough-induced chest trauma also may cause chest pain.

Pneumothorax

Spontaneous pneumothorax with attendant lung collapse stretches the pleura, causing pleuritic chest pain and dyspnea. There may be underlying emphysema, a history of prior pneumothorax, or a connective tissue abnormality such as Marfans syndrome or Ehlers-Danlos syndrome. Hyperresonance and decreased breath sounds are found on physical examination. A tension pneumothorax causes tracheal deviation, hypotension, and shock. The chest radiograph usually is diagnostic.

Pulmonary Embolism

Chest pain is a common presenting complaint among patients with pulmonary embolism.[2] Pulmonary emboli may cause localized pleuritic pain or deep, vague, substernal discomfort. Pleuritic pain is associated with smaller emboli, which cause pulmonary infarction and atelectasis. Substernal pain is more common with massive pulmonary emboli that provoke right ventricular strain, hypotension, and shock. Frequently, there is marked dyspnea, tachypnea, and tachycardia. There may be hemoptysis, a pleural rub, pleural effusion(s), low-grade fever, signs of deep venous thrombosis, or cyanosis. Risk factors for venous thromboembolism include recent surgery, immobilization, pregnancy, prior deep venous thrombosis or pulmonary embolism, oral contraceptive use, congenital or acquired thrombophilic states, and congestive heart failure.

VASCULAR CAUSES OF CHEST PAIN

Aortic Dissection

Aortic dissection may be misdiagnosed as myocardial ischemia or infarction. In addition, MI is a possible complication of aortic dissection that follows proximal (retrograde) extension to involve the coronary ostia. A diagnosis of aortic dissection is suggested by severe persistent pain radiating to the upper, interscapular, or lumbar regions of the back. It is often described as sudden, of maximal intensity at onset, and tearing, ripping, or boring in quality. There may be associated stroke, transient ischemic attacks, paralysis, ischemic limbs, gastrointestinal ischemia, and/or acute renal failure caused by compromised blood flow to vital organs.

Emphasis during the physical examination should be on the symmetry of peripheral pulses and blood pressure, the presence of aortic insufficiency, and focal neurologic findings. Signs of cardiac tamponade, which include an elevated jugular venous pressure, pulsus paradoxus, and muffled heart sounds (with traumatic tamponade), should be sought.

Aortic Aneurysm

Expansion of an aortic aneurysm can cause chest pain by erosion or impingement on nearby structures. Erosion of vertebral bodies typically causes a boring, aching, or throbbing localized pain. Common causes of aortic aneurysms include atherosclerosis, syphilis, annuloaortic ectasia, and aortic valve disease. Perforation (leaking) of an aortic aneurysm also can produce chest or back pain.

MUSCULOSKELETAL CAUSES OF CHEST PAIN

Chest Wall Pain

Musculoskeletal thoracic pain may occur in brief paroxysms (<1 minute) or persist unabating for days. It often is precipitated by abrupt movement, turning of the head or chest, or direct palpation. Unlike ischemic pain, which occurs *with* exercise, musculoskeletal pain often occurs *after* exercise and subsides slowly (hours to days).[3]

Costochondritis is a common noncardiac cause of chest pain. The discomfort is usually sharp, well localized to the costochondral or costosternal junctions, pleuritic in nature, and worsened by deep coughing or movement. There may be a history of recent strenuous or unaccustomed physical activity. The pain of costochondritis often responds to treatment with local heat, nonsteroidal antiinflammatory agents, and if necessary, injection of Xylocaine or steroids.

Tietze's syndrome, a rare cause of chest pain, is associated with swelling and erythema of the costochondral and costosternal junctions.

Rib fractures cause well-localized tenderness, usually preceded by a history of trauma, malignancy, or severe osteoporosis.

Cervical and upper thoracic osteoarthritis and herniated discs may cause chest pain with features of angina pectoris. Distinguishing characteristics of radicular pain include worsening with bending and body movement, accompanying neurologic signs and symptoms (e.g., numbness, weakness, stiffness, vertigo, tingling, paresthesias), radiation to the radial aspect of the arm or fingers, pain with coughing and sneezing, and pain with prolonged bed rest. The discomfort, at times, can be traced to a specific initiating event and elicited by rotating the head, bending the neck, hyperextending the upper spine, and applying pressure to the spine or top of the head. Plain relief frequently is obtained with cervical traction, nonsteroidal antiflammatory drugs, and analgesics; however, surgical intervention occasionally may be required if there are signs or symptoms of progressive neurologic impairment.

Thoracic outlet syndrome, including anterior scalene muscle and cervical rib syndromes, occasionally can be confused with ischemic chest pain. Compression of the brachial plexus may cause motor and sensory deficits within the ulnar distribution of the upper extremities. Obliteration of the radial pulse with the chin elevated and rotated toward the affected side (Adson's maneuver) is an important clinical finding.

Chest pain has been reported with ankylosing spondylitis, rheumatoid arthritis, psoriatic arthritis, infectious arthritis, xiphoidalgia, precordial catch syndrome (Texidors twinge), metastatic cancer, chest trauma, osteochondroma, osteosarcoma, multiple myeloma, slipping rib syndrome, and fibromyalgia.

Patients often complain of chest discomfort after open heart surgery. In addition to concerns regarding adequate revascularization and technical difficulties (involving the bypass grafts or sternal wires), other considerations include nerve entrapment, postpericardiotomy syndrome, mediastinitis, costochondritis, and superficial wound infections. Incisional chest pain often lessens in intensity over time, but may require 3 or more months to improve substantially.[4]

Herpes Zoster

Herpes zoster (shingles) can affect the anterior chest and mimic angina pectoris; however, the pain is dermatomal and does not cross the midline. Associated neurologic complaints include hyperesthesia, hypoesthesia, and dysesthesia. The pain is not relieved by nitrates or rest. The appearance of the pathognomonic vesicular rash is diagnostic, but discomfort may precede the rash by several days and in rare cases a rash never appears at all. In the elderly, posttherapeutic neuralgia is a potentially debilitating chronic chest pain syndrome.

PSYCHIATRIC CAUSES OF CHEST PAIN

Since the Civil War, chest pain has been recognized as a feature of anxiety (DaCosta's syndrome, soldier's heart, neurocirculatory asthenia).[5] The discomfort more commonly is located in the inframammary region, near the cardiac apex. It is described variably as dull and aching or sharp and stabbing. The pain can last from seconds to hours and typically is not caused by exertion but related more often to emotional strain. Associated symptoms of numbness, tingling, dizziness, perioral numbness, lightheadedness, inability to get a full breath, generalized weakness, headache, palpitations, depression, and fatigue are frequent accompanying clinical signs. Reproduction of the chest discomfort with voluntary hyperventilation may be diagnostic. The discomfort seldom is resolved without analgesics.

The patient who experiences panic attacks, hyperventilation, or depression also may complain of chest pain. In fact, up to 60% of patients with panic disorders experience noncardiac chest pain.

GASTROINTESTINAL CAUSES OF CHEST PAIN

Esophagus

Esophageal chest pain frequently is described by patients in a manner that has many features in common with angina pectoris. Among patients with chest pain and angiographically normal-appearing coronary arteries, as many as 20%–60% have an esophageal disorder.[6]

Common descriptions of esophageal chest pain include heartburn, warmth, fullness, pressure, and gnawing. The symptoms may be provoked by ingestion of food, especially at the extremes of temperature, of large quantity, or immediately after recumbency. Esophageal pain often is substernal but may extend to the right or left chest and radiate to the back. It frequently is associated with other gastrointestinal complaints, such as odynophagia, dysphasia, regurgitation, bloating, and dyspepsia. Esophageal pain can last for hours and may interrupt sleep. It can be precipitated by swallowing, exercise, or emotion and relieved by rest and nitroglycerin. The presenting history alone may not differentiate esophageal pain from cardiac pain (Table 7-1).

Gastroesophageal Reflux

Recent studies with ambulatory monitoring suggest that the most common esophageal cause of chest pain is gastroesophageal reflux. Up to 10% of patients with gastroesophageal reflux have chest pain as their only symptom. Overall, gastroesophageal reflux is found in 30%–50% of patients with noncardiac chest pain.

Esophageal Motility Disorders

Motility disorders have long been recognized as a cause of chest pain. They include "nutcracker" esophagus (high-amplitude, peristaltic contractions of long duration), diffuse esophageal spasm (frequent simultaneous contractions in the distal esophagus), lower esophageal sphincter hypertension, and achalasia.

The specific mechanisms of esophageal pain are poorly understood but thought to be mediated by chemoreceptors and mechanoreceptors.

The diagnostic studies available for evaluating patients with esophageal disorders include barium

Table 7-1. Similarities and differences between esophageal and cardiac chest pain

	Similarities of Cardiac and Esophageal Pain	Distinguishing Features of Esophageal Pain
Location	Mid or lower retrosternal. May be a severe epigastric pain with radiation to neck.	High epigastric, behind xiphoid process, or in lower retrosternal area.
Nature	Heaviness, squeezing, tightness, or burning. Can be associated with weakness, diaphoresis, and anxiety.	Often burning in nature. Heartburn is a frequent complaint. Can be associated with increased salivation and dysphagia.
Radiation	Upward toward throat. May radiate to left neck, shoulder, or arm.	Tends to ascend but not radiate to left side. Radiation to both shoulders and/or arms is less frequent. When pain begins in lower retrosternal area, it often radiates toward the epigastrium.
Precipitants	After eating. Angina is more likely with physical activity after eating.	After eating or with specific foods (alcohol, coffee, spices). Less likely to be provoked by exertion. Can be precipitated by change in posture (e.g., by lying down).
Duration	Typically brief (2–10 min.).	May last hours; typically waxes and wanes.

Table 7-1. *continued*

	Similarities of Cardiac and Esophageal Pain	*Distinguishing Features of Esophageal Pain*
Relieving factors	May be relieved by nitroglycerin, standing, and relaxing.	

Source: Modified from AJ Miller. Diagnosis of Chest Pain. New York: Raven Press, 1988;74–76.

swallow, esophagogastroduodenoscopy, resting manometry, ambulatory pH monitoring, and ambulatory manometry. Provocative maneuvers include the Bernstein acid infusion test; challenges with edrophonium, ergonovine, bethanechol, and pentagastrin; balloon distension; and ingestion of hot or cold liquids. Erosive esophagitis, hiatal hernia, and gastroesophageal reflux can be diagnosed with barium swallow and endoscopy. However, only 25% of patients with acid-related chest pain can be diagnosed with these techniques. Currently, there is no gold standard for the diagnosis of esophageal chest pain.

There are some important interactions of angina pectoris and pain of esophageal origin. Because the prevalence of both syndromes increases with age, the two may coexist. Esophageal disease has been found in up to 50% of patients with coronary disease. The mainstays of treatment for angina (nitrates, calcium channel blockers, and beta-blockers) can reduce esophageal sphincter tone, thereby worsening esophageal reflux. Similarly, these therapies can produce symptomatic improvement in patients with esophageal spasm.

Other esophageal causes of chest pain that can be severe in nature include esophageal rupture (Boerhaave's syndrome), esophageal tear (Mallory-Weiss syndrome), infectious esophagitis (e.g., herpes, candida), and irradiation-induced esophagitis.

Biliary tract disease, including sphincter of Oddi spasm, cholelithiasis, and cholecystitis, can mimic ischemic chest pain. The discomfort associated with these diseases may localize or radiate substernally and respond promptly to nitroglycerin. Furthermore, ECG changes, including ST segment elevation and depression, have been reported with biliary tract disorders.

Pancreatitis may mimic myocardial ischemia or infarction. A history of alcohol abuse or biliary tract disease may be elicited. The chest discomfort associated with pancreatitis often radiates to the epigastrium, flanks, and back.

Peptic ulcer disease can be confused with myocardial ischemic syndromes. The temporal relationship between symptom onset and either food intake or relief following antacids are important clinical features.

REFERENCES

1. Parris WC, Lin S, Frist W. Use of stellate ganglion blocks for chronic chest pain associated with primary pulmonary hypertension. Anesth Analg 1988;67:993–995.
2. Bell WR, Simon TL, DeMets DL. The clinical features of submassive and massive pulmonary emboli. Am J Med 1977;62:355–360.
3. Epstein SE, Garber LH, Borer JS. Chest wall syndrome: A common cause of unexplained chest pain. JAMA 1979;241:2793–2797.
4. Eastridge CE, Mahfood SS, Walker WA, Cole FH, Jr. Delayed chest wall pain due to sternal wire sutures. Ann Thorac Surg 1991;51:56–59.
5. Wood P. DaCosta's syndrome (or effort syndrome). Br Med J 1941;1:767.
6. Anderson KO, Dalton CB, Bradley LA, Richter JE. Stress induces alteration of esophageal pressures in healthy volunteers and non-cardiac chest pain patients. Dig Dis Sci 1989;34:83–91.

Evaluation of Chest Pain

Determining the Cause of Chest Pain

Determining the precise cause of chest pain is the primary goal of early evaluation. In this regard, the history remains the most important technique for distinguishing among the many etiologies of chest pain.[1] As a reminder, it is of utmost importance for the clinician to recognize that chest pain may originate not only in the heart but also in a variety of noncardiac intrathoracic structures including the aorta, pulmonary artery, bronchopulmonary tree, pleura, esophagus, and diaphragm, as well as subdiaphragmatic organs such as the stomach, duodenum, pancreas, and gallbladder.[2,3]

Prior to performing laboratory or other diagnostic tests it is important to fully elicit the location,

Table 8-1. Features that can be used to differentiate potential causes of chest pain

	Duration	Quality
Exertional angina	5–10 minutes	Visceral (pressure)
Rest angina	5–10 minutes	Visceral (pressure)
Mitral prolapse	Minutes to hours	Superficial (rarely visceral)
Esophageal reflux	10 minutes to 1 hour	Visceral
Esophageal spasm	5–60 minutes	Visceral
Peptic ulcer	Hours	Visceral, burning
Biliary disease	Hours	Visceral (waxes and wanes)
Cervical disc	Variable (gradually subsides)	Superficial
Hyperventilation	2–3 minutes	Visceral
Musculoskeletal	Variable	Superficial
Pulmonary	30 minutes +	Visceral (pressure)

radiation, and character of the chest pain; what precipitates and relieves the pain; the setting in which it occurs, duration, frequency and pattern; and associated symptoms (Tables 8-1 and 8-2).

Provokers	Relievers	Location
During effort or emotion	Rest, nitroglycerin	Substernal, radiates
Spontaneous	Nitroglycerin	Substernal, radiates
Spontaneous (no pattern)	Time	Sub- or parasternal
Recumbency, food	Antacids	Substernal, epigrastric
Spontaneous, cold liquids, exercise	Nitroglycerin	Substernal
Lack of food	Foods, antacids	Epigastric, substernal
Spontaneous, food	Time, analgesia	Epigastric, ± radiation
Head and neck movement	Time, analgesia	Arm, neck
Emotion, tachypnea	Stimulus removal	Substernal
Movement, palpation	Time, analgesia	Multiple sites
Activity	Rest, time, bronchodilator	Substernal

Table 8-2. Features of ischemic and nonischemic chest pain

Favors Ischemic Pain	Against Ischemic Pain
Quality of Pain	
Constricting	Dull ache
Squeezing	"Knifelike," sharp, stabbing
Burning	"Jabs" aggravated by respiration
"Heaviness," "heavy feeling"	
Location of Pain	
Substernal	Left submammary area or left hemithorax
Across mid-chest, anteriorly, both arms, shoulders, neck, cheeks, teeth, forearms, fingers, interscapular region	
Provocative Factors	
Exercise	Pain *after* completion of exercise
Excitement	Provoked by a specific body motion
Other forms of stress	
Cold weather (particularly exercise)	
After meals	

REFERENCES

1. Kleiger RE. Chest pain in patients seen in emergency clinics. JAMA 1976;236:595–597.
2. Beitman BD, Mukerji V, Lamberti JW, et al. Panic disorder in patients with chest pain and angiographically normal coronary arteries. Am J Cardiol 1989;63:1399–1403.
3. Richter JE, Bradley LA. Chest pain with normal coronary arteries: Another perspective. Dig Dis Sci 1990;35:1441–1444.

CHAPTER NINE

Life-Threatening Causes of Chest Pain

Clinicians involved in the care of patients with chest pain must be aware of several life-threatening disorders for which rapid diagnosis and treatment are imperative.[1-4] In many but not all cases, chest pain is accompanied by features of hemodynamic compromise (hypotension and hypoperfusion), hypoxia, and/or profound metabolic derangements (acid-base imbalance). A list of life-threatening causes of chest pain appears in Table 9-1.

Diagnostic benchmarks for patients with potentially life-threatening cardiovascular disorders are summarized in Table 9-2.

Table 9-1. Life-threatening causes of chest pain

- Acute myocardial infarction
- Pulmonary embolism
- Myocardial free wall rupture with tamponade (other causes of tamponade)
- Aortic dissection
- Aortic aneurysm rupture
- Tension pneumothorax
- Aortic stenosis
- Acute mitral insufficiency
- Acute ventricular septal rupture
- Esophageal rupture
- Perforated peptic ulcer
- Acute hemorrhagic pancreatitis

Table 9-2. Diagnostic benchmarks in patients with life-threatening cardiovascular disorders

	General Appearance	*Symptoms, Signs, or History*	*Jugular Venous Pressure*
Myocardial infarction	Apprehensive; cool, moist skin; agitation	Symptom onset at rest; chest pain; dyspnea; hypotension; tachycardia	↑,↔
Ventricular septal rupture	Anxious; diaphoretic	Recent MI (3–5 d);* sudden change in clinical status; chest pain; dyspnea; tachycardia	↑
Mitral insuffiency (acute)	Anxious; diaphoretic	Sudden dyspnea; recent inferior/ inferoposterior MI or history of mitral valve prolapse or history of blunt/ penetrating trauma	↑,↔

Heart Sounds	*Chest Radiograph*	*Electrocardiography*	*Other Diagnostic Tests*
S_3, S_4 gallops; ±holosystolic murmur (papillary muscle dysfunction)	Pulmonary edema	ST-segment elevation ±Q waves	Elevated creatine kinase; abnormal MB fraction (may not be elevated early); focal wall motion abnormality on echocardiogram
S_3, S_4 gallops; localized holosystolic murmur (new); palpable systolic thrill (lower left sternal border)	Pulmonary edema	Persistent ST-segment elevation; pseudonormalization of T waves; prominent U waves	L→R shunt on echocardiogram; O_2 saturation "step-up"
S_1 decreased; S_3 gallop; holosystolic murmur obscuring S_2 (A_2 component)	Pulmonary edema	Recent MI; nonspecific ST-T wave abnormality	Mitral insufficiency ± flail mitral leaflet on echocardiogram

Table 9-2. *continued*

	General Appearance	*Symptoms, Signs, or History*	*Jugular Venous Pressure*
Right ventricular infarction	Apprehensive; diaphoretic	Chest pain; nausea	↑↑
Myocarditis	Apprehensive Cool, moist skin	Viral prodrome Progressive shortness of breath; low-grade temperature; narrow pulse pressure	↑
Dilated cardiomyopathy	Diaphoretic; cool; peripheral mottling	History of chronic heart failure; narrow pulse pressure; chronic venous stasis pigmentationulceration	↑↑

Heart Sounds	*Chest Radiograph*	*Electrocardiography*	*Other Diagnostic Tests*
S_3, S_4 gallops (right side)	Clear	Inferior injury pattern with posterior extension; ≥0.5 mm ST elevation in V_3R, V_4R; bradyarrhythmias; conduction abnormalities (2°, 3° heart block)	Inferoposterior hypokinesis and right ventricular hypokinesis on echocardiogram
S_3, S_4 gallops	Pulmonary edema; heart size normal or increased	Sinus tachycardia; nonspecific ST/T changes; psuedoinfarction pattern; bundle-branch block	Chamber dilation; hypokinesis on echocardiogram
S_3, S_4 gallops; holosystolic murmur (mitral, tricuspid regurgitation)	Pulmonary edema; cardiomegaly	Sinus tachycardiaor tachyarrhythmias (atrial/ventricular); low voltage; bundle-branch block Diffuse ST/T-wave changes	Four-chamber dilation on echocardiogram

Table 9-2. *continued*

	General Appearance	*Symptoms, Signs, or History*	*Jugular Venous Pressure*
Hypertrophic cardiomyo-pathy	Anxious; diaphoretic	History of chest pain, dyspnea, syncope; family history of sudden death; apical "triple" beat; rapid carotid upstroke	↑,→ (prominent A wave)
Aortic stenosis	Pale Diaphoretic	Carotid shutter, delayed upstroke	↑
Aortic insuf-ficiency	Diaphoretic	History of hyperten-sion, endocarditis, or trauma; chest ± back pain; dysp-nea; asymmetric blood pressure/ pulses; paralysis/ sensory deficits	↑,↔
Mitral stenosis	Diaphoretic; cyanotic	Progressive dyspnea; frothy blood-tinged spu-tum; prior throm-boembolism	↑ (prominent A wave)

Heart Sounds	Chest Radiograph	Electrocardiography	Other Diagnostic Tests
Prominent S_4 gallop; holo-systolic blowing murmur at apex; holy-systolic harsh murmur left sternal border ($\uparrow$ Valsalva)	Pulmonary edema	Left ventricular hypertrophy; Q waves inferolateral leads	Septal hypertrophy on echocardiogram; out-flow tract-obstruction on Doppler studies
S_1 soft, single S_2 (P_2)	Pulmonary edema	Left ventricular hypertrophy	Aortic valve thickening; reduced leaflet motion; pressure gradient across aortic valve
S_2 soft or absent; S_2 (P_2) prominent; S_3, S_4 gallops; early, low-pitch diastolic murmur	Pulmonary edema; "calcium" sign	Nonspecific ST-T-wave changes	Aortic dissection; aortic insufficiency; trans-esophageal echocardiogram
S_1 prominent or reduced (immobile valve leaflets); P_2 prominent; opening snap; diastolic rumbling murmur	Pulmonary edema; right ventricular prominence; left atrial enlargement	Tachyarrythmia (particularly atrial fibrillation); right-axis deviation; right ventricular hypertrophy; atrial enlargement	Calcified, stenotic mitral valve

Table 9-2. *continued*

	General Appearance	*Symptoms, Signs, or History*	*Jugular Venous Pressure*
Pulmonary embolism	Anxious; cyanotic	Sudden pleuritic chest pain, dyspnea, cough, hemoptysis, or syncope; risk factors for pulmonary embolism; tachypnea (>20 breaths/min)	↑ (prominent A wave)
Cardiac tamponade	Pale; anxious; apprehensive	Hypotension; narrow pulse pressure; distended neck veins; pulsus paradoxus	↑↑ (absent Y descent)

Heart Sounds	Chest Radiograph	Electrocardiography	Other Diagnostic Tests
Distant (rapid accumulation of pericardial fluid); ± friction rub	Normal or enlarged cardiac silhouette	Low voltage; T-wave flattening	Pericardial effusion; right atrial, right ventricular collapse on echocardiogram; abnormal Doppler flow patterns

*May occur earlier (24–48 hours) following fibrinolytic therapy.
L→R = left to right; MI = myocardial infarction; P_2 = pulmonic second heart sound; S_1 = first heart sound; S_2 = second heart sound; S_3 = third heart sound; S_4 = fourth heart sound; ↔ = normal; ↑ = increased; ↑↑ = markedly increased.

REFERENCES

1. Snell RJ, Parrillo JE. Cardiovascular dysfunction in septic shock. Chest 1991;99:1000–1009.
2. Page DL, Caufield JB, Kastor JA, et al. Myocardial changes associated with cardiogenic shock. N Engl J Med 1971;285:133–137.
3. Parker MM, McCarthy KE, Ognibene FP, Parrillo JE. Right ventricular dysfunction and dilatation, similar to left ventricular changes, characterize the cardiac depression of septic shock in humans. Chest 1990;97:126–131.
4. Abraham E. Host defense abnormalities after hemorrhage, trauma, and burns. Crit Care Med 1989;17:934–939.

Diagnosing Ischemic Chest Pain

Individuals with suspected ischemic chest pain must be evaluated expeditiously for several reasons. First, myocardial ischemia, if prolonged and severe, can cause myocardial necrosis (infarction). Second, treatment strategies are widely available for patients with acute coronary syndromes (unstable angina, non-ST-segment elevation MI, ST-segment elevation/bundle branch block MI) that reduce morbidity and mortality. Third, the overall impact of treatment and the benefits derived are most profound with early intervention.[1–3]

ELECTROCARDIOGRAPHIC FINDINGS

The electrocardiographic (ECG) hallmarks of myocardial ischemia are ST-segment depression and changes in T waves (Figure 10-1A). Significant ST-segment depression is present when the ST-segment measures >1 mm (0.1 mV) below the PT-baseline at the J-point. The J-point of the ECG is defined as the angle between the end of the QRS complex and the start of the ST segment. The ST segment can be upsloping (often a nonspecific finding), horizontal (more specific for ischemia), or downsloping (most specific for ischemia).

The T-wave changes of ischemia, in general, are less specific and consist of either T-wave inversion (relative to the axis of the QRS complex) or T waves that are tall, peaked, and symmetrical. Giant, "hyperacute" T-wave changes, at times, are the only electrocardiographic changes seen in the early stages of MI. Dynamic deep T-wave inversions involving two or more anatomically contiguous leads, when present, are highly suggestive of myocardial ischemia.

Some nonischemic clinical conditions that can cause ST-segment depression and T-wave changes are left ventricular hypertrophy, early repolarization, complete left bundle branch block, ventricular preexcitation (Wolffe-Parkinson-White syndrome), and digitalis.

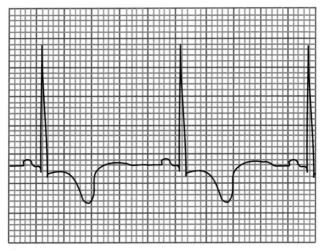

A

Figure 10-1. ECG findings. (A) The ECG features of myocardial ischemia include deep and symmetric T-wave inversions and ST segment depression. The latter feature offers greater specificity, particularly if the changes are dynamic in nature.

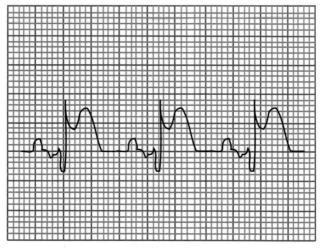

B

Figure 10-1. *continued* (B) The ECG hallmark of myocardial injury is convex upward ST-segment elevation in two or more anatomically contiguous leads.

MYOCARDIAL INJURY

Myocardial injury occurs when there is a critical reduction in blood flow for a prolonged period of time. For myocyte death to occur, total occlusion of a coronary artery usually is required for 20–40 minutes.

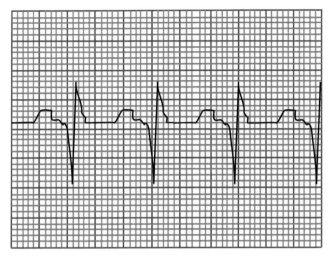

C

Figure 10-1. *continued* (C) Myocardial necrosis (infarction) is associated with pathologic Q waves (>40 msec wide, ≥25% height, of R wave). The only exception is seen in posterior myocardial infarction that causes prominent R waves (R:S>1) in the early precordial leads (V_1–V_3).

The likelihood of injury is facilitated by the absence of a well-developed collateral circulation.

The ECG hallmark of myocardial injury is convex upward ST-segment elevation (Figure 10-1B). ST-segment elevation is significant when the

ST-segment measures ≥1 mm (calibration = 0.1 mV/1.0 mm) above the PT-baseline at a point 0.06 seconds beyond the J-point. In general, the greater the degree of ST-segment elevation and the greater the number of involved ECG leads, the greater is the specificity (and extent) of myocardial injury.

MYOCARDIAL INFARCTION

The term *myocardial infarction* (MI) refers to the actual death of injured myocardial cells. Myocardial injury can progress to infarction within minutes to hours. With death, the myocardial cells lose cell wall integrity. Intracellular components such as creatine phosphokinase (CK), troponins, and myoglobin begin to leak out into the bloodstream. They then can be measured as serum markers of MI.

The ECG hallmark of myocardial necrosis is the presence of Q waves (Figure 10-1C). Q waves are considered abnormal if they are ≥1 mm (0.04 sec) wide with a depth of greater than 25% of the height of the R wave that follows in the same lead. An exception to the rule is observed with posterior MI, where prominent R waves (R:S>1) are present in the early precordial leads (V_1–V_3).

Q waves represent infarcted myocardial tissue and can appear within hours of complete coronary occlusion, but usually no less than 2 hours after symptom onset. The presence of Q waves, appreciated in the absence of acute clinical signs and symptoms, supports a prior infarction; however, the Q-wave appearance provides no information on when the event took place. When considered in the context of ST- and T-wave morphology, an approximation of timing usually can be made.

Although the surface ECG can appear entirely normal in patients experiencing an acute MI, certain diagnostic features should be familiar to all clinicians, given their importance in management and, ultimately, in patient outcome. To be considered significant, ECG changes should be seen in two or more anatomically contiguous leads. An acute injury pattern, corresponding to a specific coronary anatomic distribution (Table 10-1) is supported by a convex upward ST-segment elevation of ≥1.0 mm (0.1 mV) in the standard (I, II, III) and augmented (aVF, aVL) leads and ≥2.0 mm (0.2 mV) in the precordial leads. An exception is acute posterior wall injury, where horizontal ST-segment depression with upright T waves is seen. When suspicion for injury is high, posterior leads (V_7, V_8, V_9) should be performed. Right ventricular infarction is heralded

Table 10-1. Anatomic and electrocardiographic correlations in myocardial injury or infarction

Leads with ECG Changes	Injury/Infarct-Related Artery	Area of Damage
V_1–V_2	LAD-septal	Septum; His bundle; bundle branches
V_3–V_4	LAD-diagonal	Anterior wall LV
V_5–V_6	Left-circumflex	Low lateral wall LV
I, aVL	LAD-diagonal branch	High lateral wall LV
II, III, aVF	RCA-posterior descending	Inferior wall LV; posterior wall LV
V_4R (II, III, aVF)	RCA-proximal branch	RV; inferior wall LV; posterior wall LV
V_1–V_4 (marked depression)	Either left circumflex or RCA posterior descending	Posterior wall LV

LAD = left anterior descending artery; RCA = right coronary artery; LV = left ventricle; RV = right ventricle.

by the presence of ≥0.5 mm (0.05 mV) ST-segment elevation in leads V_3R or V_4R.

Several examples of acute myocardial injury and infarction patterns appear in Figures 10-2 through 10-5.

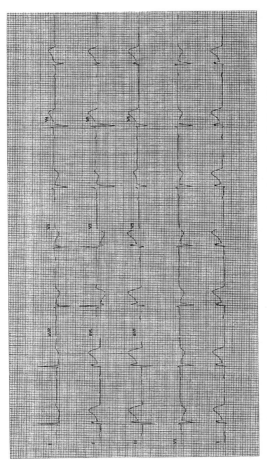

Figure 10-2. Acute myocardial injury pattern involving the inferior (II, III, aVF) and lower-lateral or apical (V$_5$, V$_6$) walls.

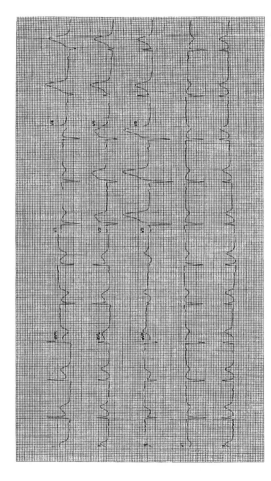

Figure 10-3. Acute myocardial injury pattern involving the anterior (V_1–V_6) and high-lateral (I, aVL) walls. Evidence of infarction (Q waves) is seen in leads V_1–V_4.

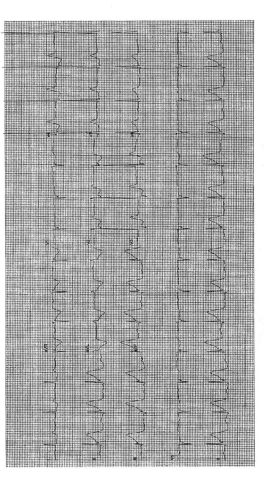

Figure 10-4. Acute myocardial injury pattern invoking the inferior (II, III, aVF) wall. Posterior wall involvement is evident with horizontal ST-segment depression with accompanying upright T waves in leads V_1–V_4.

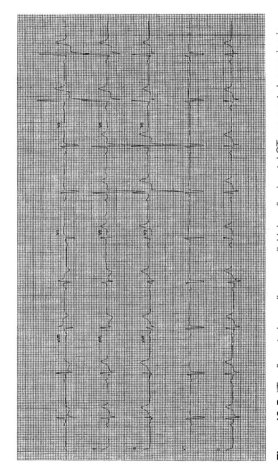

Figure 10-5. "True" posterior wall myocardial injury (horizontal ST-segment depression in leads V_3–V_6).

REFERENCES

1. Goldman L, Weinberg M, Weisberg MC, et al. A computer derived protocol to aid in the diagnosis of emergency room patients with acute chest pain. N Engl J Med 1982;307:588–596.
2. Christie LG, Conti CR. Systematic approach to evaluation of angina-like chest pain: Pathophysiology and clinical testing with emphasis on objective documentation of myocardial ischemia. Am Heart J 1981;102:897–912.
3. McCarthy BD, Wong JB, Selker HP. Detecting acute cardiac ischemia in the emergency department: A review of the literature. J Gen Intern Med 1990;5:365–373.

CHAPTER ELEVEN

Identifying High-Risk Patients

Patients with myocardial ischemia and acute coronary syndromes can be triaged (risk stratified) into risk categories based on a combination of demographic, historic, clinical, and ECG features. Patients at greatest risk for MI and cardiovascular death or those with either dynamic ST-segment changes, persistent ST-segment elevation, or signs of hemodynamic compromise (hypotension, congestive heart failure, shock; see Table 11-1). These patients require prompt intervention.[1–3]

Table 11-1. Risk of death or nonfatal MI for patients with ischemic chest pain

High Risk (at least one of the following)	Intermediate Risk (no high-risk features plus one of the following)	Low Risk (no high- or intermediate-risk features plus one of the following)
Prolonged continuing pain not relieved by rest	Prolonged angina but resolved at time of evaluation ("stuttering")	Angina—increased in frequency, severity, or duration
Pulmonary edema S_3 or rales	Rest angina lasting >20 min or relieved with nitroglycerin	Lower activity threshold before angina
Hypotension with angina	Age >65 years	New-onset angina >2 wk to 2 mo prior
Dynamic ST changes >1 mm	Dynamic T-wave changes Q waves with ST deviation ≥1 mm	Normal or unchanged ECG

Source: Modified from U.S. Department of Health Care Services; 1994. AHCPR Publication No.: 94-0602.

REFERENCES

1. Becker RC, Grella RD. Cardiogenic shock complicating coronary artery disease: diagnosis, treatment, and management. Curr Prob Cardiol 1994;19:693–744.
2. Becker RC, Burns M, Gore JM, et al. for the National Registry of Myocardial Infarction (NRMI-2) Participants. Early assessment and in-hospital management of patients with acute myocardial infarction at increased risk for adverse outcomes: A nationwide perspective of current clinical practice. Am Heart J 1998;135:786–796.
3. Berger PB, Holmes DR, Stebbin AL for the GUSTO-1 Investigators. Impact of an aggressive invasive catheterization and revascularization strategy on mortality in patients with cardiogenic shock in the GUSTO-1 trial. Circulation 1997;96:122–127.

PART FOUR

Management of Ischemic Chest Pain

CHAPTER TWELVE

Immediate General Treatment

Hospital-based management of patients with ischemic chest pain should follow the American Heart Association's recommended clinical pathway.[1] The four therapies currently include:

1. Oxygen (4L/min).
2. Nitroglycerin (sublingual or IV; if systolic blood pressure >90 mmHg).
3. Morphine sulfate (1–3 mg IV at 5-min intervals).
4. Aspirin (325 mg as a starting dose; clopidogrel 300 mg starting dose for patients allergic to aspirin).

The recommendations apply to each subset of patients experiencing an acute coronary syndrome. It is important to emphasize the importance of maintaining perfusion pressure in patients with obstructive coronary artery disease. In this context, nitroglycerin and morphine should be used cautiously when there is hypotension or evidence of right ventricular infarction.

Every emergency department should establish a protocol or clinical pathway for patients with ischemic chest pain and suspected MI. This facilitates consistency in patient care and provides a mechanism for documenting the outcome.

Clinicians practicing in an ambulatory setting also must have guidelines for the management of patients with ischemic chest pain. Measurement of vital signs (including oxygen saturation), attachment of a cardiac monitor, establishing peripheral venous access, and alerting the emergency medical services system are important initial steps. Aspirin, nitroglycerin, and oxygen should be provided; however, it is vital that transport to the nearest emergency department not be delayed.

REFERENCE

1. American Heart Association. Advanced Cardiac Life Support Manual. Dallas, TX: American Heart Association, 1997–1999.

CHAPTER THIRTEEN

Immediate Targeted Therapy

The rapid assessment of patients with suspected ischemic chest pain, as outlined in Chapter 10, should include a surface 12-lead ECG and determination of overall risk based on an established triaging score (Figure 13-1).

The 12-lead ECG represents the pivotal tool for both early diagnosis and management of acute MI. Patients with either ST-segment elevation or a new bundle branch block are known to benefit from immediate reperfusion therapy, either in the form of fibrinolytics or primary coronary angioplasty. Thus, a careful review and interpretation by an experienced clinician must take place promptly.[1–3]

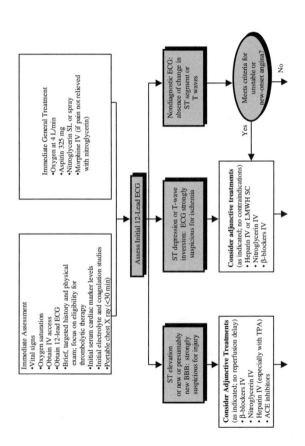

Immediate Assessment
•Vital signs
•Oxygen saturation
•Obtain IV access
•Obtain 12-lead ECG
•Brief, targeted history and physical
 exam; focus on eligibility for
 thrombolytic therapy
•Initial serum cardiac marker levels
•Initial electrolyte and coagulation studies
•Portable chest X ray (<30 min)

Immediate General Treatment
•Oxygen at 4 L/min
•Aspirin 325 mg
•Nitroglycerin SL or spray
•Morphine IV (if pain not relieved
 with nitroglycerin)

Assess Initial 12-Lead ECG

ST elevation
or new or presumably
new BBB: strongly
suspicious for injury

ST depression or T-wave
inversion: ECG strongly
suspicious for ischemia

Nondiagnostic ECG:
absence of change in
ST segment or
T waves

Meets criteria for
unstable or
new-onset angina?

No

Yes

Consider Adjunctive Treatments
(as indicated; no reperfusion delay)
• β-blockers IV
• Nitroglycerin IV
• Heparin IV (especially with TPA)
• ACE inhibitors

Consider adjunctive treatments
(as indicated; no contraindications)
• Heparin IV or LMWH SC
• Nitroglycerin IV
• β-blockers IV

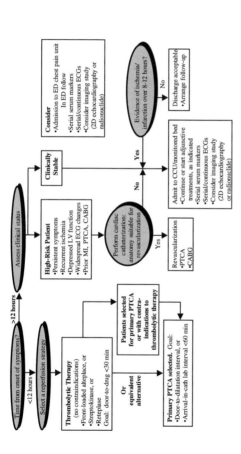

Figure 13-1. Management algorithm for patients with ischemic chest pain. A key initial step determines the presence (or absence) of acute myocardial injury and the need for immediate reperfusion therapy (fibrinolysis or primary coronary angioplasty). (Modified from Ryan TJ, Anderson JL, Antman EM, et al. American College of Cardiology/American Heart Association guidelines for the management of patients with acute myocardial infarction. A report of the American College of Cardiology/American Heart Association Task Force on Practice Guidelines [Committee on Management of Acute Myocardial Infarction]. J Am Coll Cardiol 1996;28:1328–1428.)

ADJUNCTIVE PHARMACOLOGIC THERAPY

Patients with acute ischemic chest pain (acute coronary syndrome), in addition to the treatment strategies outlined in Chapter 12, should be considered for adjunctive therapy that includes:

1. Beta-blockers
2. Calcium channel antagonists (when beta-blockers are either contraindicated or have failed to suppress symptoms completely)
3. Heparin (unfractionated or low molecular weight)
4. Angiotensin-converting enzyme (ACE) inhibitors

In the setting of acute ST-segment-elevation MI, it is important to emphasize that reperfusion therapy must not be delayed in favor of adjunctive agents. Instead, clinicians should view adjunctive therapy as a means to supplement definitive treatment by reducing oxygen demand (beta-blockers, nitrates), improving oxygen supply (calcium channel antagonists), stabilizing atheromatous plaques and improving vascular endothelial cell function (ACE inhibitors), preventing thrombotic coronary arterial reocclusion (aspirin/heparin) and attenuating maladaptive myocardial remodeling (ACE inhibitors). To achieve these important goals, adjunctive therapy should be introduced within the first 24 hours when clinically feasible.

Patients with unstable angina and non-ST-segment-elevation MI do not benefit from reperfusion therapy; however, they should receive general and targeted treatment as previously outlined. In addition, high-risk patients should be considered for treatment with a platelet glycoprotein (GP) IIb/IIIa receptor antagonist. There are currently three FDA-approved intravenous agents. Abciximab (ReoPro®), eptifibatide (Integrilin®) and tirofiban (Aggrastat®). Intravenous GPIIb/IIIa receptor antagonists may also be beneficial in patients with ST segment elevation MI where they can be used conjunctively with low-dose fibrinolytics or primary coronary interventions.

REFERENCES

1. Ryan TJ, Anderson JL, Antman EM, et al. American College of Cardiology/American Heart Association guidelines for the management of patients with acute myocardial infarction. A report of the American College of Cardiology/American Heart Association Task Force on Practice Guidelines

(Committee on Management of Acute Myocardial Infarction). J Am Coll Cardiol 1996;28:1328–1428.

2. American College of Cardiology/American Heart Association Task Force on Practice Guidelines (Committee on Management of Acute Myocardial Infarction). 1999 Update: Guidelines for the management of patients with acute myocardial infarction. J Am Coll Cardiol 1999;34:890–911.

3. Braunwald E, Mark DB, Jones RH, et al. Unstable Angina: Diagnosis and Management. Clinical Practice Guideline Number 10. Rockville, MD: Agency for Health Care Policy and Research and the National Heart, Lung, and Blood Institute, Public Health Service, U.S. Department of Health and Human Services; 1994. AHCPR Publication No.: 94-0602.

CHAPTER FOURTEEN

Chronic Management Guidelines

Ischemic heart disease remains a major health problem and, in a majority of cases, chronic stable angina is the initial manifestation. The American Heart Association has estimated that 6.2 million Americans have ischemic chest pain. Indeed, despite a documented decline in cardiovascular mortality, ischemic heart disease remains the leading cause of death and is responsible for 1 of every 4.8 deaths.[1–5]

The clinical assessment of patients with chronic chest pain applies specifically to clinicians practicing in an ambulatory setting and guidelines, as proposed by the American Heart Association, American College of Cardiology, and American College of Physicians,[6] are designed to identify patients with

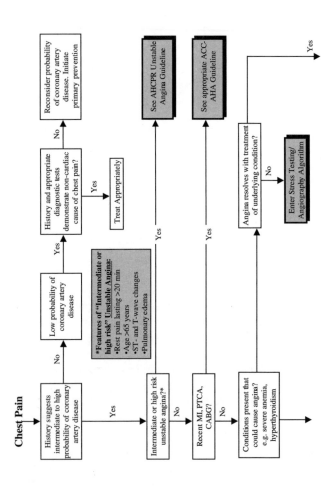

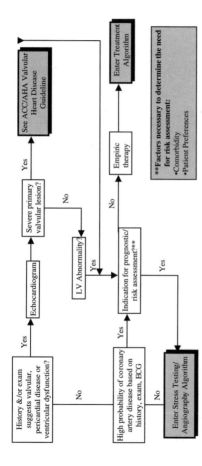

Figure 14-1. Chest pain management algorithm designed to identify patients with acute myocardial ischemia and those at risk for myocardial infarction and cardiac death. AHCPR = Agency for Health Care Policy and Research; MI = myocardial infarction; PTCA = percutaneous transluminal coronary angioplasty; CABG = coronary artery bypass graft; ACC = American College of Cardiology; AHA = American Heart Association; LV = left ventricular; and ECG = electrocardiogram. (Adapted with permission from Gibbons R. Guidelines Chronic Stable Angina. J Am Coll Cardiol 1999;33:2092–2197.)

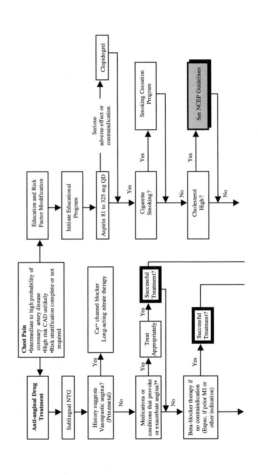

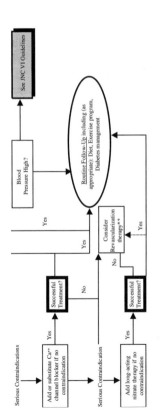

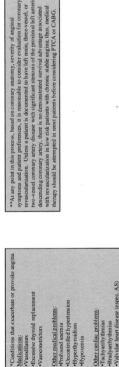

*Conditions that exacerbate or provoke angina
Medications:
 • Vasodilators
 • Excessive thyroid replacement
 • Vasoconstrictors

Other medical problems:
 • Profound anemia
 • Uncontrolled hypertension
 • Hyperthyroidism
 • Hypoxemia

Other cardiac problems:
 • Tachyarrhythmias
 • Bradyarrhythmias
 • Valvular heart disease (espec. AS)
 • Hypertrophic cardiomyopathy

**At any point in this process, based on coronary anatomy, severity of anginal symptoms and patient preferences, it is reasonable to consider evaluation for coronary revascularization. Unless a patient is documented to have left main, three-vessel, or two-vessel coronary artery disease with significant stenosis of the proximal left anterior descending coronary artery, there is no demonstrated survival advantage associated with revascularization in low risk patients with chronic stable angina; thus, medical therapy should be attempted in most patients before considering PTCA or CABG.

Figure 14-2. Chronic chest pain management algorithm that addresses both risk factor modification and pharmacologic treatment. (Adapted with permission from Gibbons R. Guidelines Chronic Stable Angina. J Am Coll Cardiol 1999;33:2092.)

underlying ischemic heart disease and those at high risk for cardiac events (Figure 14-1).

The treatment of chronic ischemic chest pain has two complementary objectives: (1) to reduce symptoms and improve quality of life and (2) to reduce the risk of myocardial infarction and cardiovascular death. Initial treatment measures should include:

1. Aspirin and antianginal therapy.
2. Beta-blocker and blood pressure control.
3. Cessation of cigarette smoking and reduction of cholesterol.
4. A heart-healthy diet and diabetes control.
5. Education regarding heart disease, risk factors, and regular exercise.

A comprehensive treatment algorithm has been proposed (Figure 14-2). All patients with chronic ischemic chest pain also should receive a prescription for sublingual nitroglycerin, education in its proper use, and instruction on the indications for emergency medical services.

REFERENCES

1. Kannel WB, Feinleib M. Natural history of angina pectoris in the Framingham study. Prognosis and survival. Am J Cardiol 1972;29:154–163.

2. The American Heart Association. 1999 Heart and Stroke Statistical Update. Dallas, TX: American Heart Association, 1999.

3. The American Heart Association. Biostatistical Fact Sheets. 1997. Dallas, TX: American Heart Association, 1997;1–29.

4. National Cholesterol Education Program. Second Report of the Expert Panel on Detection, Evaluation, and Treatment of High Blood Cholesterol in Adults (Adult Treatment Panel II). Circulation 1994;89:1333–1445.

5. 27th Bethesda Conference. Matching the intensity of risk factor management with the hazard for coronary disease events. September 14–15, 1995. J Am Coll Cardiol 1996;27:957–1047.

6. Gibbons R. Guidelines Chronic Stable Angina. J Am Coll Cardiol 1999;33:2092–2197.

PART FIVE

Case Studies

Case Studies

PSYCHIATRIC CAUSE OF CHEST PAIN

A 50-year-old man is referred to the Cardiovascular Clinic for evaluation of chest pain of 8 years duration. His symptoms began 4 months after the death of a family member and are described as sharp and variable in provocation, location, and intensity.

GASTROINTESTINAL CAUSE OF CHEST PAIN (GASTROESOPHAGEAL REFLUX)

A 40-year-old woman complains of intermittent epigastric discomfort that is described as burning in quality with radiation to the mid-chest and throat.

The symptoms, lasting 20–40 minutes, most often occur after meals but occasionally at night, awakening her from sleep. Several recent episodes were accompanied by a bitter taste in her mouth.

PULMONARY CAUSE OF CHEST PAIN (ACUTE PULMONARY EMBOLISM)

A 35-year-old man is admitted to the Intensive Care Unit for evaluation of chest pain. He has been recovering from arthroscopic surgery that took place 5 days earlier. His symptoms began suddenly and were accompanied immediately by shortness of breath. The pain, poorly localized across the anterior chest, is worsened with inspiration. His respirations are labored, and he is markedly diaphoretic.

VASCULAR CAUSE OF CHEST PAIN (ACUTE AORTIC DISSECTION)

A 70-year-old man with long-standing suboptimally controlled systemic hypertension is brought to the emergency room by his wife for evaluation of sudden onset, severe, substernal chest pain radiating between the shoulder blades to the lower back. The symptoms began suddenly and have been unremitting for the past hour. His presenting blood pressure is 240/120 mmHg in the right arm and 200/80 mmHg in the left arm.

MUSCULOSKELETAL CAUSE OF CHEST PAIN

A 38-year-old man has experienced recurrent episodes of sharp, stabbing, well-localized left parasternal chest pain over the past 6 months. His symptoms occur both at rest and following exertion, lasting from seconds to hours in duration. Twisting movements and deep inspiration worsen the pain.

ISCHEMIC CHEST PAIN—UNSTABLE ANGINA

A 65-year-old man with hypertension and hypercholesterolemia presents to the Emergency Department with substernal chest pressure radiating to the neck and left shoulder. Similar episodes have occurred with decreasing levels of exertion over the past few days, typically lasting between 5 and 10 minutes. He became concerned when symptoms appeared at rest.

ISCHEMIC CHEST PAIN—ACUTE
MYOCARDIAL INFARCTION

A 58-year-old woman with diabetes mellitus, hypertension, and a 30-pack/year smoking history is brought to the Primary Care Clinic for evaluation of nausea, vomiting, diaphoresis, and interscapular back pain. Her symptoms began 12 hours prior to presentation, waxing and waning initially, but over the past 2 hours have been unremitting.

ISCHEMIC CHEST PAIN—CHRONIC
STABLE ANGINA

A 75-year-old man with borderline systemic hypertension and a 3.5 cm abdominal aortic aneurysm is seen in clinic for a yearly physical examination. He offers a complaint of chest burning and mild shortness of breath over the past 6–8 months that predictably begins 10–15 minutes into his daily walk. Both symptoms lessen as he continues; however, upon further questioning it is apparent that he has slowed the pace of his walking and changed the route to avoid several inclines and hills.

NONISCHEMIC CARDIAC CHEST PAIN—ACUTE PERICARDITIS

A 25-year-old woman is evaluated in the Urgent Care Clinic for chest pain and shortness of breath. She had been seen several weeks earlier with complaints of fever, cough, and nasal congestion. The chest pain is described as sharp, localized to the left sternal border, and worse with coughing, swallowing, and lying flat. Her respirations appear rapid, shallow, and "splinted."

Index